A Teenager's Perspective on Food Restrictions: A Practical Guide to Keep from Going Crazy

Erica Brahan

~To my mom~
Thank you for continuously taking the time to
support me through this journey,
always caring, and never giving up hope.

~To my dad~
Thank you for always going with the flow
and being willing to try new things.

~To Hanna~
Thanks for always listening and encouraging me
through every step in this journey.

"He must become greater; I must become less."
John 3:30

To God be the glory.

TABLE OF CONTENTS

{INTRODUCTION}

This book will not tell you how to regain your health but it will offer advice for any teenager who is considering changing their diet for health reasons or who already have food restrictions. This book is simply a reflection of my experiences and what I have learned. I do not pretend to have all the answers or to have everything figured out, because this journey is a constant learning and growing experience.

The advice offered is also not very specific because of how different your situation could be from mine. Our journeys aren't going to be the same, and you may not agree with my opinions because of our different experiences. That is fine. Regardless, I hope this book encourages you to keep going through your journey as much as writing it has for me.

{MY STORY}

Since I was very young, I have had health problems, but they seemed unrelated until a few years ago. When I was around six months old, I had my first ear infection. Between the ages of two and three, I had constant ear infections that would not go away.

Three sets of ear tubes/vents were put in to try to stop my eardrums from rupturing. Then my adenoids were removed. During this time, I was on continuous antibiotics.

The older I got, the more sensitive to foods and the environment I seemed to become. I was lactose intolerant and sensitive to pollen, dust, and strawberry and bean plants. My family did countless rounds of allergy treatments that helped temporarily, but didn't fix the root of the problem. There was always a new sensitivity appearing.

The first time I can remember my joints and muscles bothering me was in fourth grade after I sprained my ankle. I wore ankle braces after that to provide extra support when I played sports, but there was still discomfort. From there the joint inflammation only spiraled downward.

I started playing softball when I was six years old. I fell in love with the sport and catching, but the countless days I spent squatting took a toll on my knees. In seventh grade, I started wearing knee braces in hopes they would eliminate the pain, but they didn't. The joint inflammation spread, so more joints were affected and the pain intensified as I got older.

Going into my freshman year of high school, I was training for cross-country and catching up to eight games a week. By the end of the summer, I couldn't walk without pain and catching was almost unbearable. I ended up trading in cross-country for four months of physical therapy for my knees. The muscles around my knees were strengthened, but the therapy didn't eliminate the joint pain.

Shortly after this, a rapidly growing large, gray yeast rash appeared on my neck. I was told it wasn't a big deal and not to worry. This was the first time I began to question if something bigger was going on.

Around this time, I also began to deal with deep, painful cystic acne[1] and weight gain. I started having typical teenage acne in seventh grade, but just like with the joint pain, the older I got, the more out of control it became. The weight was almost unexplainable; after all, I was eating well and active. It felt like no matter what I did, I had no control over my body. Everything continued to worsen.

The summer going into my sophomore year of high school was almost worse than the summer before. At the end of two back-to-back softball seasons, I developed tendonitis[2] in both knees and elbows, multiple fingers, left wrist, and right bicep. My forearms burned from what felt like constant sore muscles. My fingers felt stiff and hurt to bend. I couldn't lift my arm to my shoulder without a deep stabbing pain. It was relentless and got worse with activity.

My mom offered to take me to her functional medicine doctor[3] to examine my arm and to start to identify the cause of the tendonitis. I went reluctantly, not wanting to make the diet changes my mom had. I had no more patience to deal with the spreading tendonitis and just wanted answers, because I was finally realizing it wasn't normal or a result of my catching.

This is when my journey of healing began.

During the beginning of sophomore year, at 15 years old, I was taken off of gluten, dairy, corn, MSG, sugar, and soy and began taking additional supplements. I saw small improvements in acne and joint pain. Although the joint inflammation improved briefly, I still was experiencing discomfort and pain often. During that softball season, I had two chiropractic adjustments a week, but the adjustments did not hold because of the inflammation. Later, I developed an intense stabbing sensation in both my feet and the other symptoms remained with little improvement.

Searching for more answers to my family's health issues, my mom began the GAPS diet[4] during fall of my junior year. My brother was going to be starting it as well, so I joined them, with the approval of my doctor, as a way to support my brother. I knew it would help me, because I was learning that a poorly functioning gut, Leaky Gut Syndrome[5], results in countless symptoms, one being chronic joint inflammation. I began to see improvements in acne and joint pain again, and to my relief, the pain in my feet disappeared completely. The new diet was working, but it was not enough. I still had many other symptoms such as stretch marks on my legs, cracking joints, weight gain, thick mucus in my throat, and poor lymph circulation.

I learned I had developed a sensitivity to salicylates[6], and my doctor instructed me to remove all foods with moderate to high levels of salicylates that spring. By removing salicylates from my diet, my body began to release what it had stored. I could only eat around 20 foods, but within a month, *all* the joint pain was gone for the first time in five years.

The joint inflammation has not returned, but the cystic acne still flares up, the weight continues to increase, and I struggle to detox.

My mom has persistently researched for more answers and came to the conclusion to have a genetic test and a complete metabolic blood test conducted. The genetic test revealed two mutations with my MTHFR gene[7]. The blood test was used to confirm that these genetic mutations are affecting my body as a whole and my liver's ability to detox.

As of now, April 2014, I am working diligently to support my liver and to stop the gene from expressing itself. I am doing this through exercise supplements, and following a limited diet with the help and guidance of my mom and doctor.

{REALITY}

The purpose of this chapter is not to frighten you and cause you to not follow your diet, but rather to give you a heads up of what you may go through. How difficult this journey will be is different for everyone, but there will be challenges. No one told me about the problems a restrictive diet would bring. So, that is what this is- the warning I wished I received. Don't get overwhelmed and think you won't be able to handle this though, because you can.

If you choose to read this chapter, then you have to finish reading the rest of the book. Although there are many negatives, the positives that come from changing your diet will far outweigh the challenges.

WHY DIET RESTRICTIONS ARE PARTICULARY HARD FOR TEENS

Although a struggle for nearly everyone regardless of age, adjusting to and managing any type of issue with food seems to be particularly hard for kids, teens, and young adults.

The first reason for this struggle is that regaining your health and life requires that a variety of character traits be developed, including:

* Self-Control
* Maturity
* Commitment
* Motivation
* Discipline
* Gratitude
* Perseverance
* Responsibility
* The ability to overcome disappointment

In general, people don't like change, so without the traits listed above change can be hard to adjust to. It is normal to not want to give up your favorite foods because that requires change.

When first changing your diet, there is often the mental boundary that the removal of foods is harder than it really is. I hear, "How can you do that? I could never give that up!" It is a lot of work to heal your digestive systems. Perseverance and commitment are necessary.

There are additional factors I believe make teenagers less inclined to agree to change their diets:

* Wanting to fit in
* Lacking support from peers
* Not wanting to "lose" their social life
* Rearranging priorities and time commitments
* Difficulty associated with the persistence

Again, the majority of these factors also affect adults but they are magnified in teenagers.

When eating anything but the standard American diet, teens stand out and may be labeled as different or not normal. When you don't fit in there is typically a desire to find others like you, but there is not usually a very strong and united support system for teens with food restrictions.

Finally, food restrictions not only affect your lives right now but also decisions about the future (discussed later). If the health problem isn't urgent or affecting daily living, then it can be easier to ignore it than ponder its future effect. Additionally, teens do not always think beyond instant gratification, so it can be difficult to recognize the future benefits when a change in your health may not be noticeable for days, weeks, and even months.

Although challenging, it is more than possible for you to change your diet as a teenager. There are many things fighting for your attention: friends, sports, media, work, health, family, and school, to name a few. If you are willing to rearrange your priorities, put in the work, and try to have a positive attitude, anything is possible.

REALITY CHECK

You go from being a normal-ish teenager, as normal as any teen can be that is, to being labeled as kind of weird. Your friends will try to understand, but it is hard for them. They will offer you food you can't eat, even though you have explained it many times.

There is not a lot of support to be offered. It can be lonely. It's likely your group of friends is not going through what you are, and you might not meet anyone who is.

Having a social life can be difficult at times. Events often include food, and if you don't bring your own food or eat before, you have to ask about ingredients or read labels. Ingredients you can't eat will show up in foods and even hygiene products you never thought to check. Giving up little things like a food you really like can be harder to give up than an entire food group.

There is temptation everywhere, and it can consume your thoughts when you are around food you can't have. It's easy to sneak a bite when no one is looking. Food becomes scary; even though you want to reintroduce foods on an elimination diet, it is scary waiting to see if you are going to react. It can get very frustrating. Sometimes, you take one step forward and then take two steps back. Progress won't happen at the pace you want, and even steps forward don't feel good enough, because you're still far away from the end.

There are times you may feel so overwhelmed, stressed, and hopeless that you just want to cry—all you want to do is quit. You might be angry that you were given these health problems and angry you aren't normal.

And here is the kicker: you *will* mess up.

After reading many of the negatives that come with food restrictions, it is hard to imagine why anyone would choose to do this if they don't have to. Getting your health back takes time and effort. It can be long, frustrating, lonely, and definitely not easy, but it is worth it. It's okay that you're not normal. Who wants to be a stereotypical teen? You learn what foods are and aren't allowed and eventually just know what not to eat. Setting goals (discussed later) helps with overcoming temptation. You will find friends who do their best to support you and accommodate your diet. Although it's more difficult, you can still have a social life. If you are on an elimination diet, you regain foods at the pace your body can handle. There are times of great accomplishments and improvements.

Yet, don't forget, perfection is an unattainable myth. It's okay to mess up as long as you don't give up.

{MOTIVATION}

Restrictive Restrictions

The Merriam-Webster dictionary defines restriction as, "the act of limiting or controlling something," and two synonyms provided are "constraint" and "limitation." I would like to challenge the common idea that food restrictions bring restrictions into our lives.

By avoiding certain foods or following an elimination diet, you are getting back your health. You are freeing yourself from feeling sick. You are giving up foods that are harming your body and are instead taking in foods that will nourish your body, which is the purpose of eating.

You may be prevented from doing certain activities and feel like it is your food restrictions, not your health, holding you back, but think about what you are gaining. The benefits far outweigh what you are giving up. By addressing these issues and changing the way you eat, you are gaining freedom and a brighter future in the long-term. In a nutshell, food restrictions bring freedom not limitations.

Try creating your own definition of food restrictions (page 85).

IT'S A MARATHON NOT A SPRINT

You now have your own definition of food restrictions and possibly a new perspective, but sadly this doesn't help your body heal any faster. It's cliché but true; elimination diets and food restrictions are a marathon, not a sprint.

This may not always seem fair, and it can be a struggle to stay focused and patient while you wait for your body to heal, but keep in mind that your body is more complex than ever imaginable. Every gene, hormone, and organ is connected and interwoven, and directly or indirectly affect each other. When one part fails to function properly, another is quick to follow and rebel.

As you begin to address your health issues, it may be straightforward and easy, but there is also the chance that it's not going to be as easy as it seems. As you fix one health problem you might discover another part of your body isn't working to its potential that you weren't able to see before because of how dominant the other one was.

A good analogy of this is peeling an onion. An onion has many layers and in order to get to the core, you have to keep pulling back those layers. The same goes for your body. You have to peel away one issue at a time, until the root of your health problems are exposed.

Your body doesn't work on your time though, so wellness can feel like an eternity away. Every time you make the choice to eat a food that will help your body rather than harm it, you are taking a step forward. It may be a tiny step, but it is still a step forward. You may not see it in the moment but every one those little steps count and add up into leaps and bounds of improvements and progress that you can see only when you look back.

DREAMS AND GOALS

There are three important questions you should ask yourself before changing your diet.

1. Why am I doing this?

_____

_____

_____

_____

_____

_____

Answer this question honestly, and try to put aside the reasons your parents or anyone else has. This is your journey, not theirs—so why are *you* doing this? When you take ownership of your health, you are more willing to follow your diet restrictions, because you know why *you* are choosing to eat this way.

28

2. What are my dreams? Is my current health preventing me from achieving them?

_____

_____

_____

_____

_____

_____

_____

_____

Think about what you want out of changing your diet: to be healthy? If so, then, elaborate. What specifically do you want?

Your dreams don't have to be exactly food-related either. For example, my dreams have been to decrease the chance of passing my health issues to my future children, to travel more conveniently, and to not be concerned if my health will prevent me from living my life to the fullest.

It is important to distinguish the difference between goals and dreams though. A dream is something you desire and the end result that drives your actions. Goals, on the other hand, are what it takes to achieve your dream. Dreams are just that, dreams. Goals require action. Focus on your dream, but work on achieving your short and long-term goals to make your dream a reality.

3. What goals are needed to achieve my dream? What steps do I need to take to reach those goals and ultimately my dreams?

Once you figure out your dreams and goals, write them down and put them somewhere you can see daily. If you are feeling creative or are more of a visual person, create a dream board to represent your dreams. After you do this, share your goals. Talk to family members and friends. Pick a friend to hold you accountable for your diet. It is easier to ignore your food restrictions when there is no one asking you about them. Figure out what is needed to accomplish your goals and rearrange your priorities to make them happen.

Set a timeline for your goals. Remember though, your body doesn't work on *your* time. Don't be disappointed if progress is slower than you expect. It can be slow. Don't lose hope, because that is when you lose motivation. Hold on to and celebrate the small steps forward. There will be setbacks and moments when you want to quit, but that's when you remember your dreams and reasons for creating a healthier life for yourself. Your attitude shapes your actions. Remember that every day brings you one day closer to regaining your health and reaching your dreams.

You are doing this at a young and difficult age, but your age is also an advantage. You are actively doing something to improve your health before it worsens and causes more problems in the future. Some people will deal with health problems their entire lives, but you can chose to not let yours spiral out of control. Although it can be hard to see, everything you are doing is helping. It is a short-term loss of foods for the long-term gain of health and freedom. The reward of reaching your goals and being healthy will be longer than the journey getting there.

When Health Overpowers Happiness

It is easy to feel weighed down by every ailment and treatment, which can cause your stress levels to go crazy. The more stressed out you are, often the worse your health becomes. This is a dangerous cycle you can get caught in quickly.

If you are feeling overwhelmed, mentally exhausted, or simply stressed out, here are four tips that may help you get out of the cycle.

1. **Remember your dreams.**
    When things get hard, remember why you changed your diet and what you are fighting for. When there seems to be no near end to the marathon, remember what is waiting for you at the finish line.

2. **Take a breath.**
    Panicking doesn't help the situation, and it only will cause more stress. Everything will work out. Maybe not the way you want, but it will work out, and you will be able to handle it. Try to calm down, focus on breathing, and not worry about the worst-case scenario. Being terrified about

what could happen before it does is not how you want to live, because it will put you in a negative state-of-mind.

3. **Let it go.**

There are times you don't have control over your body. You can manage your stress, eat right, get enough sleep, and exercise but still not feel well. Although your body is not the enemy, it is failing you. It can become an impossible burden to carry if you blame yourself for every symptom or day you don't feel well. Keep doing what you know and research what else might help.

4. **Laugh.**

Being so uptight and stressed that you can't enjoy what is right in front of you is no way to go through life. Spend time with the people who will make you laugh and get your mind off your health for a while. Don't be afraid to laugh at yourself either! Sometimes it's best to look at your situation and find the humor in it.

{SOCIAL LIFE}

Planning

There are many social opportunities teens have, such as, hanging out with friends, vacations, eating out, parties, sports, and weekend retreats. How do you avoid living in an isolated bubble and still effectively managing food?

Planning is essential. You will no longer be able to go with the flow and eat whatever, whenever. When you run out of food, it is time to go home. Planning ahead helps with this. Every time you leave your house for an extended period of time, you need to consider whether you need to bring food. This can be tedious but necessary if you still want to be socially active.

Depending on the severity of your food restrictions, eating out or at other people's houses may not be possible. You will need to think ahead about what and when to eat. Depending on the event, it can be easier to eat ahead of time. If you are comfortable with how you eat, pack your own food. If you aren't comfortable eating in front of others but need to bring food, pack something that is more 'normal'.

If your food restrictions are not as tight and you are going out to eat, search for the restaurant online and see if they have posted a menu. Call the restaurant if you have more questions. Chain restaurants often post menus and ingredient lists for customers like you. If you have more specific questions for chain restaurants, email the company and they will help you.

Encourage your friends to go places you know you can eat at ahead of time.

If you don't want to go out, for whatever reason, then don't. Watching others eat what you can't isn't exactly fun, but you can choose if you're going let it bother you or not. Decide what you would rather do, spend time with friends and family watching them eat but still have fun or stay home. The choice is up to you; don't let friends pressure you into a situation involving food that you don't feel comfortable in. It becomes easier to watch others eat, still not fun, but easier at least. Don't let food control your decisions; if it's important to you, then try to make it work.

There will be events you really cannot go to though, even if it is important to you. In these situations, you need to decide what is more important, attending or your health and goals. You need to make responsible and mature decisions that your body will thank you for, even when you don't want to. Regaining your health needs to come before your social life in order to reach your goals.

Diet restrictions are not a death sentence to your social life. If you make mature and responsible decisions and plan ahead, you will still be able to go on vacations, spend time with friends and family, play sports, go to parties, and be involved in extracurricular activities.

DATING

Before starting a relationship with another person beyond friendship, whether it is casual or serious, it would be good for that person to know about your food restrictions. Like it or not, your food restrictions are part of what makes you unique, so be upfront about it, because there is nothing to be ashamed of.

Relationships require honesty and this includes your food restrictions. When you first start dating, it is not necessary to go into every detail of your medical history. If you see the relationship progressing into something more serious and long-term, then it will need to be discussed, especially if you have a more serious health issue. If your boyfriend or girlfriend cannot support and handle what you are going through, then that person is not the right person for you.

I overheard two girls talking once about a friend of theirs who is lactose intolerant and went on a date. They were saying how horrible it would be if the guy had planned a date and it was ruined, because he didn't know she couldn't eat dairy. They continued to say they couldn't imagine dating without meeting at coffee shops and going out for ice cream.

Try to be creative about ideas for dates. Social gatherings often involve food, and dating is not excluded. Think outside of the box for activities that don't involve food but would still be fun and build your relationship. If you do want to eat together, pick a restaurant ahead of time you know is safe or cook together at someone's house. Cooking together is a good way to meet the person's parents while introducing them to your favorite recipes and way of eating.

If you have an anaphylaxis allergy, the guidelines to dating are more detailed and rigorous. Please do more research before you start dating, so you are well prepared.

TRUE FRIENDS DON'T CARE?

Yep, you read that right. True friends don't care.

They care about you, but they don't care about what you eat. Let me try to explain...

I hated eating my weird food in front of people—I still do at times. I would eat before I went somewhere or come home hungry, because I didn't want to eat around people I didn't know. If I had to bring food some place, I avoided sitting close to people and hid my food, so I wouldn't have to answer questions. One day it just hit me. Why do I care what people think of me just because of the way I eat?

I realized I really shouldn't care. The people who truly care about me as a person just want me to be healthy. They don't care that I bring meatball and squash soup in a thermos for lunch or a bowl of cold peas as a snack. They accept that part of me.

Does that mean that your friends will understand everything you are going through? No, of course not. They probably won't, but that doesn't stop them from supporting and encouraging you. A true friend may not understand everything, but he or she will do his or her best to understand. Of course, your friends are going to mess up and do things like offer you food you can't eat. Be patient with them. They are not perfect. None of us are, but they are trying.

41

This may be hard to hear, but if your friends aren't even trying to be supportive or are making fun of you because of the way you eat, you need to either talk with them to see what's going on or think about making new friends. Being around people who judge you and only see you for your health issues and food restrictions drags you and your attitude down. None of this is constructive in working towards your dreams while also meeting your goals.

When you are in a group of strangers it can be difficult, since you stick out for the way you eat. It may feel like they are staring at you or your food, which is possible, but there is also a good chance you are making it into a bigger deal than it really is. Remember who is important to you, and do your best to get through the situation.

This idea is applicable to many parts of your life, not just your health. The people who are important to you don't care, or care a lot less about what you eat, wear, look like, or do. They care about you as a person, not about the outward appearance.

EXPLAINING YOUR REALITY

Explaining why you cannot eat like the people around you can feel embarrassing and intimidating. It might take a little time before you figure out a good way to explain to others why you don't eat what they do, but you will figure it out, and it will become easier. In most situations, keep your explanation short. It's not that the people asking don't care; it's just that they probably were not expecting a five-minute response and might not understand all of it. You don't need to explain the whole situation. Don't lie. If you are embarrassed or feel like it would be too difficult or frustrating to explain, don't.

Here are a few things to say when avoiding a long explanation:

* "I don't eat _____."
* "I can't eat _____ because of health reasons. It's not a big deal."
* "I'm allergic (or sensitive) to _____."
* "I would just rather eat what I packed."
* "_____ doesn't make me feel good."

There. Done. They know enough that if they want to ask more questions, they can. Give a simple explanation, and you might be surprised by how supportive people will try to be.

When you are struggling mentally or emotionally to understand why you have these health problems, it is less desirable to explain what's wrong with you. It is normal to get frustrated and annoyed with the questions though. You still get to choose your attitude when you respond to the questions. Your friends are asking because they care about you or are curious. Give a respectful answer, because you never know how you can inspire others.

{GOING TO SCHOOL}

School Days

Going to school with food restrictions can make some aspects more difficult, but it is possible in the majority of cases. An invaluable piece of advice to remember whenever you go to school, or anywhere really, is that you can choose whose opinions matter to you.

As discussed earlier, your true friends do not care what you eat. They just want you to be well. When you have a group of friends, who have a basic understanding of what you are going through, then it is easier to eat at school, especially during lunch. Anyone who makes a rude or mean comment about what you are eating should be ignored. Their opinions only matter if you let them.

Lunches and snacks are tricky depending on your food restrictions and the school's rules. If you are allowed to eat in class, bring foods you are comfortable eating in front of others. If you are not allowed to eat in class, leave a snack ready in your locker so you can grab it and go. If there is nothing you are able to bring to school as a snack, eat a bigger breakfast, so you are not as hungry by lunch. When possible, prepare your lunches and snacks the night before (discussed next).

Another challenging situation in school are food-orientated class periods or events. The worst part is watching everyone eat and not participating. It would easy to sneak a bite and eat, but it's not worth it if you want to reach your goals. Yes, the food will taste good for a short time, but it also can leave you feeling sick and regretful. Saying no to food offered to you becomes easier. Once it becomes habit to say no, it is less tempting to say yes, because you think about it less.

SAVE TIME IN THE MORNING

Unlike many of your peers, you likely have to actually cook your food in the morning, and this takes time. Be grateful for the food and cooking. Yes, they take up some of your time, but you are on your way to be becoming healthier, and that is something you can be grateful for. A positive attitude has the potential to make a huge difference in the morning.

Here are three tips on how to save time:

1. **Eat "non-breakfast" foods.**
   There's no rule saying, "For breakfast you must eat pancakes, cereal, or toast." Eat whatever is most practical for you and your diet. If having soup or warming up a hamburger with vegetables is the quickest or easiest for you, then do that. Leftovers are also practical for breakfast; they are easy to warm up and require little attention.

2. **Make food in large quantities.**
   When you make a recipe, double or even triple it and put the extras into the fridge or freezer for longer storage. This is referred to as batch cooking. If you are on an elimination diet and storing food in the freezer, write down the ingredients on the bag or on a piece of tape on the

container. This is helpful if you have to remove additional foods from your diet and want to know quickly what ingredients were used.

Cooking food in large quantities not only saves time in the morning, but it also makes cooking easier. Instead of making the same recipe three times and making three times the mess, you will only have to gather the ingredients and clean dishes once.

3.   **Prepare breakfast and lunch the night before.**
Think about what you are going to eat the night before. Is it already made or do you have to cook it in the morning? Do you have to take it out of the freezer? This changes how much time you need to eat and cook in the morning. When preparing lunches, place the food you want into containers the night before. This helps speed up the process in the morning, because it will be ready to go in containers and only needs to be packed and possibly warmed up. In addition to being good for breakfast, leftovers are good for lunches, because they require little to no additional cooking.

PREPARATION FOR SCHOOL LUNCHES

My creativity tends to be lacking when it comes to packing lunches and snacks at school. I bring the same few foods over and over, which is fine, because I know what does and doesn't work.

There are six items that I highly recommend owning if you are a kid with food restrictions and attending school. These items are not only beneficial for school, but also for anytime you are packing food. Most of these are probably obvious and you may already own them, but a few may be new to you.

1. **Lunch Box.**

    As a kid with limited food options, you probably have to pack a lot of your own food. When you are bringing a whole meal or food that needs to stay a certain temperature, then it would be a good idea to use a lunch box. It will get a lot of use, so purchase one that you like.

2. **Thermos.**

    Seriously, I love my thermoses. They are good for anytime you want to keep your food warm or cold for a long period of time. I would recommend buying a high quality stainless steel one, because they are more difficult to break and do not contain the harmful chemicals that are found in plastic thermoses. Most thermoses also come with a collapsible spoon making traveling easy and convenient.

3. **Water Bottle.**

Water is vital for our bodies, and if your school allows it, you should be drinking water during the day. Fill your water bottle before school and make it a goal to drink it all by the end of the school day.

4. **Containers.**

Using containers over zipper bags is more economical in the long run because they are reusable. They are good for packing foods that are liquidly, and they also prevent squashing your food.

5. **Ice Packs.**

You most likely already have at least one ice pack and know the benefits of owning one, but here it is anyways. They help keep food that needs to stay cold, like meat, cold for long periods of time. If your food is at the temperature you prefer, in this case cold, then it is more desirable to eat.

6. Spork.

Please agree with me on this one, otherwise I'm probably sounding pretty weird. I think these are really neat. I mean, come on! It's a fork, knife, and spoon all in one! This is not a necessity, but I just think it is cool and convenient for traveling.

{OTHER ADVICE}

NORMAL PEOPLE LIVE NORMAL LIVES

When you eat differently than people around you, you naturally stand out, which isn't always a bad thing. A mentor of mine had the unfortunate opportunity of listening to me say "I just want to be normal and eat like everyone else". She turned that statement around by asking what being normal meant to me. I responded by saying that being normal means I don't stand out. Then she said something I have yet to forget, "Normal people live normal lives, and you have no desire to have an ordinary life."

You really only have two options: go through the motions of life and merely exist or stand out and accomplish your dreams. If your desire to be normal is so strong it prevents you from living your life, then think back to those dreams. You probably have huge dreams you want to achieve during your life, most of which won't happen unless you take risks, change your health, and stand out. If you don't want to just exist, then why do you want to be normal? It doesn't make any sense!

By not being normal, you may also have some amazing opportunities to share your story and what you are going through. Every struggle you have can be learned from and turned into something positive that can inspire and help others. You never know the impact your story, actions, and attitude will have.

Wanting to be normal isn't wrong; it's pretty natural to want to fit in. This desire doesn't go away until your attitude and actions change, until your desire for something else is bigger than your desire to be normal. What is it that you want? Focus on that consistently, and you will find that not being normal is worth it!

TODAY I CHOOSE TO BE HEALTHY

When each day is a struggle to have a good attitude, say to yourself, "Today I choose to be healthy because..." This is a way to remind yourself what you are working towards or what your goals are.

Try this next time you are feeling sorry for yourself. You might be amazed how much this saying can help! Make a list of all your reasons, so when you have a really bad day, you can look back at it and be reminded of all your reasons for changing your diet (page 85).

Have a positive outlook about your circumstances. Being negative doesn't help, and it only makes you and the people around you miserable. Life is rough; you didn't ask for these health problems, but you are actively doing something to change your health for the better. Your health isn't your identity, and it doesn't determine your worth as a person. Hold on to each baby step and success rather than the setbacks and disappointments that might come your way.

THERE IS A REASON

I believe everything has a plan and a purpose. Although, it is often difficult to see in the moment, there is a reason you are going through this. It is very possible you don't even have a clue yet as to what that reason is, but there is one. There will be periods of unavoidable hardship in our lives but each has a purpose.

"I have said these things to you, that in me you may
have peace. In the world you will have tribulation.
But take heart; I have overcome the world."
John 16:33 (ESV)

There are many, many lessons to be learned from food restrictions and elimination diets, but you need to have your eyes open to see them. Whatever that reason is, it is all meaningful and important.

Choosing A College

When selecting a college, there are several factors to consider depending on the severity of your restrictions:

1.   Do I need to cook my own food, and will I have access to a kitchen?

2.   If I am consulting with a medical professional, will I still have a way to be in contact with him or her?

3.   Are there any safe food options on campus?

4.   Are the food plans mandatory or are they flexible?

5.   Is there a program or a coordinator to help accommodate my dietary needs, if necessary?

6.   Do I have access to purchase foods I need off campus?

You may find that some of these do not apply to you, or that there are more questions to be asked, but it is very important to consider how college will affect your health. Think through each college option carefully and thoroughly. For some, this will include whether or not leaving home and living on campus is a beneficial decision to your immediate and long-term health.

Tiny Tidbits

* **Poison to Your Body:**
Food that is harmful to your body needs to be looked at as a poison. You need to stay as far away from foods that aren't beneficial. Eat as cleanly as possible whenever you can.

* **It's Okay to Mess Up:**
Not that you want to make a habit of it, but it's okay to mess up every now and then. Don't beat yourself up over a mistake, because no one is perfect. Pick yourself up and keep doing the best that you can.

* **Family Support:**
Food restrictions are easier when your family is eating similarly. Encourage at least one member of your family to eat like you. They will be able to offer support and help you with cooking.

* **Make a Daily Checklist:**
Remembering everything you have to do or not do in a day can be overwhelming. Creating a checklist of reminders is helpful and holds you accountable for your

actions. Also, it can help you remember everything until it becomes a habit.

✴ **Don't Cut Everything Out Right Away:**
If you are nervous about changing your diet and don't know what recipes you'll eat, start slowly. Don't stall too long though, because the sooner you start, the sooner you can begin to feel better.

✴ **New Foods or Recipes:**
There is a good chance the foods you loved before diet restrictions are no longer allowed. Start looking for new recipes. The Internet is your new best friend for this. Keep folders or bookmarks of the recipes you like on your computer or print them to store in a binder. Either way, having them organized makes the cooking go faster.

Not all the recipes you make have to be new. Try modifying the recipes you already enjoy eating. You can look online to find a version of the recipe that fits with your diet or you can look up substitutions for specific ingredients.

✴ **Picky Eaters:**
Try the food. Don't rule it out right away; at least, have a bite and then decide if you like it or not. You might be surprised by how your taste buds change as your diet changes.

* **Keep a Logbook:**
  If you are on an elimination diet, get a notebook and track what you are eating on a day-to-day basis. Experiment until you find a system that works for you, whether that means writing everything down at one time or every time, you eat.

  Also, write down how you feel or symptoms you have during that day. This is a good way to hold yourself accountable for what you are eating and also to track how what you eat affects your body. Only do this if you think it would be helpful though, because it has the potential to be stressful.

{OTHER TEEN STORIES}

COLIN

14 years old
I eat a healthy and restrictive diet
that is similar to the GAPS diet.

I was born the eighth out of nine children in a loving family who, for many years, lived in Illinois, and then approximately a year after I was born, we moved to Colorado for my father's writing job. I grew up there, loving the winter with the constant blankets of snow and the clouds giving a warm feeling inside.

And yet, there was still a problem that we paid no mind to. There was something there that we now wished we had paid attention to. It wasn't until I was seven years of age when everything began to crumble slowly, surely, and sadly.

I was diagnosed in late July 2007. Those two and a half days in the hospital were days I'll never forget.

Of course, at first, I knew not what the disease was, only that from here on out, it was going to be a whole lot harder.

It was a disease called Type 1 Diabetes[8].

Not too long after, we located what had caused this disease—stachybotrys; a black mold that decimated our livelihood and health.

For eight years, it had eaten at us, and the many, many visits to the doctor clearly displayed it to us.

Then, November 2008, we left.

I went through the front door, got into the car, excited to sleepover at someone's house for the first time, not knowing I was seeing mine for the last time.

In the morning, my parents broke the news. We were not going back home.

For the next week or so, we lived out of a couple of hotel rooms, with extremely few possessions. I had a couple of action figures, a few pairs of clothes, and only the memory of two dogs that I never got to say goodbye to.

And then, I moved on.

We rented a house in Colorado, and near Christmas time, we moved out to Arizona.

"Why Arizona?" I once asked my mom.

She replied by saying we were out there to see a mold doctor. He would have answers, which was all we were looking for at the time.

Then, over a long and financially exhausting period, we finally were able to see past the steam on the mirror and realize what was staring at us right in the face. It wasn't the heaps of medications and prescriptions that would help and nourish our bodies. It was the simple and plain fact the whole world tends to cover up: food is what heals.

I had to find this fact out the hard way, and it definitely was not easy. We first began on GAPS, and the first day was the hardest. Twenty-four hours of just soup.

I was starving the whole day. The next day, I found that I could surprisingly limit my intake of food without a problem.

Slowly, over the course of the next five years or so, we began to get healthier. My blood sugars slowly began to stabilize, my A1C was the best doctors had seen in a long time, and they were utterly befuddled as to the cause, and likewise my Lantus dosage went down to record lows.

We continually kept making changes to our eating lifestyle. We took out foods, like rice, fruit, regular store-bought yogurt and milk, cereal (even the healthy kind), peanut butter, crackers, *any* junk food whatsoever, and a multitude of other things I loved back then.

But we would also add certain foods.

We later brought fruit back in and were able to replace quinoa with rice. While I was improving, it also plainly showed in other parts of the family. Tempers were not as flared as they once were; tension slowly began to decrease. Rashes mysteriously disappeared, and to have a cold or get sick was unheard of for at least six months.

Of course, the doctors were utterly shocked as to why we were improving so much. Yet, we continued to get better. I'm not saying that dieting or eating healthy is the answer to everything, but it's not that far off from the truth.

We continue to eat this way and get healthier.

Wednesday is one of my favorite days of the week, because I get raw milk, a bag of frozen fruit, and almond butter to ferment overnight, and cream for either whipped cream or to use it to make almond cookies. Many days, I will make stir-fries, often with salmon.

Every day, I am continually encouraged that I am *constantly* getting better. I love to go to the gym and to come home and make a smoothie. I can't believe how good sauerkraut sounds to me now or how much I enjoy having avocado ice cream.

Although I may face many more challenges ahead of me, I know they can be conquered, and I know that I will push through. The food I eat will keep me going. *The food I eat will help me conquer the challenges, even if the challenge itself is food.*

JUSTIN

13 Years Old
Specific Carbohydrate Diet (SCD)[9]

I have had a problem in the past with eating foods that are not part of my restrictive diet.

I am 13 and have Crohn's Disease[10].

I have been on SCD for three years now. I'm not suppose to eat foods not on my diet, and as long as I follow my diet strictly, I am symptom and medication free.

It was very hard when I was home alone or out with friends to not eat foods that are not on my diet. I think it was a struggle for me because of the fact that I can't have certain foods, which makes them taste that much better and makes me want to have them that much more. In one sense, it was kind of addictive to be craving to eat foods not on my diet. The foods didn't make my stomach hurt, but they made me feel achy all of the time and prevented me from being active, the one thing I love to do.

So, I got myself a ring that I wear every day with a Bible verse on it to remind me that I have the strength to say no to those foods, because God gives it to me. I just have to use that strength. Ever since I started wearing my ring, I have felt so much better, because I am not cheating and have been able to practice basketball all day, everyday, and have still felt good. I am still sore from just being active, but it is much better than when I was eating foods I wasn't supposed to.

{Conclusion}

You might be at the point where you can't stand your parents for making you eat this way. Maybe you are angry and bitter that you have to deal with this and would rather ignore your health problems. Maybe you know what makes you sick, but you still eat it and deny its affects. Maybe you don't fall under any of these categories.

If you are dealing with health problems as a teenager, then you didn't have to read this book to know how hard it can be, but I hope you've learned that your age is an advantage when it comes to food restrictions and elimination diets. By confronting these issues now, you are preventing them from getting out of control. You've now learned a few strategies for how to deal with situations that could come your way. Most importantly, you've learned that the short-term losses are worth the long-term gains.

Just knowing these things isn't enough—it is time to step up. No more whining, complaining, and expecting others to do everything for you. It is your body, not your parents', not your doctors'—*yours*. This means you need to take responsibility for it. You can take responsibility for your health by researching to understand what you are going through, being motivated, following your diet, helping with cooking, and having a positive attitude. You want to be healthy? You want to achieve those goals? Then it is time to step up and take responsibility for your health.

You can say you are only a teenager or still a kid, but that's no longer an excuse. You are old enough to understand consequences, see the big picture, and the future you are heading towards. Some day, you will move out your house and won't have parents around to monitor everything you do and eat. It will be completely on you to make smart and responsible decisions. Your parents' desire for you to live a healthy life is not enough. You have to want it and be willing to work for it. Making good choices now will help to create a healthy lifestyle when you are on your own. Your attitude shapes your actions, and if you have a positive attitude and take responsibility for your health, then your journey will truly be *your* journey.

My personal journey is not over. Progress has been slow and difficult, but I have no regrets. Is this journey hard? Definitely. Is it worth it? Definitely! I would not go back and change my decision to do this. I would do it all over again just for the lessons I have learned and the progress I have made. I feel the best I have in five years, and I have no more joint pain and that relief, besides my dreams and goals, is what keeps me motivated.

It is your body, your health, and your life – not anyone else's, so take responsibility. Don't forget, it gets easier; it is okay not to be normal, and it is all definitely worth it.

{RECIPES}

Coconut StrApple Bars

Ingredients:
* 1 cup thawed or fresh strawberries
* 2 cups shredded apples
* 1 cup shredded coconut
* 1/4 cup melted coconut oil
* 1 T. honey (optional)

Special Equipment:
* Dehydrator
* Food Processor or Blender

Directions:
1. Place the strawberries, apples, and honey into the food processor or blender
2. In a small bowl, pour the coconut oil on top of the shredded coconut and mix briefly. Add this combination to the rest of the ingredients.
3. Blend the ingredients together until all the fruit chunks are gone.
4. Spread evenly on to a dehydrator pan, approximately 1/4 inch thick.
5. Dehydrate at 135°F for 4 to 5 hours. It is done when it is hard enough to hold together but is not brittle.

6.   Cut into square portions and store in the refrigerator.

To view the images of this recipe, please visit
http://edibleattitudes.com/bookrecipes/

Dairy-Free Banana Mango Ice Cream

Makes about 2 ½ cups

Ingredients:
* 1 frozen banana
* 2 cups frozen mangos
* 1/3 cup coconut milk
* 1 tsp. gelatin (optional)

Special Equipment:
* Food Processor or Blender

Directions:
1. Place the fruit into the food processor or blender and let it thaw for 10 minutes
2. Combine the coconut milk and gelatin with the fruit.
3. Blend together until there are no fruit chunks.

Note:

✳   If the fruit is not blending quickly or the coconut milk is thick, continue to add one tablespoon of coconut milk at a time until the fruit moves easier in the blender.

✳   The ice cream can be frozen, but it is better fresh.

To view the images of this recipe, please visit

http://edibleattitudes.com/bookrecipes/

{GLOSSARY}

1. **Cystic Acne:** A severe case of inflammatory acne where deep skin tissue is affected. Large, long-lasting and painful acne occurs.

2. **Tendonitis:** A condition where tendons become inflamed, irritated, or swollen.

3. **Functional Medicine Doctor:** A practitioner who looks at the interconnected systems of our body then uses foods, supplements, and other therapies to address the root cause of health issues rather than treating symptoms.

4. **Gut and Psychology Syndrome (GAPS) Diet:** An elimination diet protocol put together by Dr. Natasha Campbell-McBride to help heal the gut. The recommended foods are eggs, meat, nuts, and a lot of healthy fats. Certain fresh fruits and vegetables are also permitted.

5. **Leaky Gut Syndrome:** A condition when the lining of the small intestine becomes compromised (gets holes in it), and food particles leak from the small intestine into the bloodstream leading possible immune reactions to foods.

6. **Salicylates:** One of many naturally occurring chemicals in food that function as a natural pesticide.

7. **MTHFR:** Methylenetetrahydrofolate Reductase is a gene that is part of methylation and can affect the body's detox pathways.

8. **Type 1 Diabetes:** An autoimmune disease that is also known as juvenile diabetes where the pancreas cannot produce insulin to remove glucose from the blood.

9. **Specific Carbohydrate Diet (SCD):** Protocol for healing the digestive system and body through eating foods such as select meats, vegetables, fruits, nuts, legumes, and dairy products.

10. **Crohn's Disease:** An autoimmune disease that occurs when the body creates an immune system response and begins attacking the gastrointestinal tract causing chronic inflammation.

Looking for a community to connect with?
Visit edibleattitudes.com

Or join the Teens with Food
Restrictions Facebook group!

TODAY I CHOOSE TO BE HEALTHY BECAUSE...

1. _____

_____

2. _____

_____

3. _____

_____

4. _____

_____

5. _____

_____

FOOD RESTRICTIONS ARE...

_____

_____

_____